# YOUR JOURNEY TO HEALTH AND FITNESS

## GENERAL TIPS

## KATE .P

# Contents

# CHAPTER ONE

## INTRODUCTION

"Your Journey to Health and Fitness" is a life-changing journey that touches on every facet of your being rather than just a goal. It's a wholistic approach to wellbeing that puts equal emphasis on mental and physical health and strives for long-term lifestyle adjustments as opposed to band-aid solutions.

Starting this path entails making a commitment to your well-being and future, understanding that genuine health extends beyond outward appearances and scale readings. It's about being alive, invigorated, and self-assured in your own flesh.

Understanding and self-awareness are the first steps in this path. Consider your present routines, both good and bad, and note where you may make changes. Whether your objective is to be happier and more balanced or to gain strength, improve flexibility, or lose weight, make sure your goals are reasonable and in line with your values and aspirations.

In every path toward health and fitness, nutrition is essential. For best results and overall wellbeing, fuel your body with foods that promote your objectives. Instead of rigid deprivation, aim for balance and moderation while concentrating on complete, nutrient-dense diets.

Another essential component of a healthy lifestyle is physical activity. Choose enjoyable pursuits that provide your body with a variety of challenges, such as strength training, aerobics, yoga, or outdoor excursions. Make activity a regular component of your regimen; consistency is crucial.

However, fitness and wellness go beyond the physical. Developing an optimistic outlook, successfully handling stress, and placing self-care first are all equally crucial components of your path. Engage in mindfulness exercises, surround yourself with encouraging people, and don't be scared to ask for expert assistance when necessary.

Recall that your path to fitness and health is personal to you. Accept the highs and lows, acknowledge your accomplishments, and draw lessons from failures. Along the journey, remember to be curious, dedicated, and most importantly, kind to yourself. If you put in the effort and don't give up, you'll not only accomplish your goals but also feel empowered and full of life outside of the gym.

## Characterizing Fitness and Health

Fitness and health are multifaceted ideas that include different facets of mental, emotional, and physical well-being. Despite their close relationship, their foci are slightly different:

Health: A state of total well-being that includes social, mental, and physical components is referred to as health. It encompasses more than just the absence of illness or disability; it also refers to qualities like vigor, fortitude, and the capacity to overcome obstacles in life. A healthy individual has a high degree of functional capacity and is able to participate completely in everyday activities.

Contrarily, fitness is particularly concerned with physical characteristics and abilities linked to function and performance. It consists of elements including flexibility, muscular strength and endurance, cardiovascular endurance, and body composition. Targeted physical activity and training are usually required to improve fitness, which is commonly assessed through a variety of tests and evaluations.

Fitness and health are two different but closely related concepts. Improving fitness levels is generally necessary to get optimal health because a healthy lifestyle must include both appropriate nutrition and regular physical activity. On the other hand, physical fitness can improve general health by lowering the risk of chronic illnesses, improving mental health, and increasing lifespan.

In the end, fitness and health are dynamic processes requiring constant work, dedication, and balance. A meaningful and sustainable lifestyle requires aiming for a holistic approach that takes mental and physical health into account.

## Goal-setting and Self-Assessment

Setting goals and doing a self-evaluation are essential first stages in starting and maintaining a path toward fitness and health. Here's a methodical technique to get you going:

Self-Evaluation:

Physical Health: Take into account your weight, body measurements, cardiovascular endurance, muscular strength, flexibility, and any current medical issues while assessing your present physical health.

Nutrition: Consider your eating patterns. Think about the kinds of foods you usually eat, how much you eat at each meal, when you eat it, how hydrated you are, and any dietary requirements or limitations you may have.

Mental and Emotional Well-Being: Evaluate your general mental health, stress levels, mood, and sleep quality. Consider how these things affect your day-to-day activities and capacity to achieve your fitness and health objectives.

Lifestyle Practices: Consider your sleeping habits, sedentary activity, drug use (such as drinking alcohol or smoking), and screen time. Determine which areas require improvements that could improve your overall health.

Motivation and Readiness for Change: Think about the reasons you are starting this journey and the obstacles or difficulties you could encounter. Evaluate your dedication to putting your health and fitness first and your readiness to undertake lifestyle changes.

Establishing Objectives:

Specificity: Clearly define your objectives and the outcomes you hope to attain. Clearly state your goals, whether they be to run a marathon, lose a specific amount of weight, or increase your general fitness.

Measurability: To monitor your development over time, make sure your objectives are quantifiable. Make use of quantitative measures like weight loss, growth in inches, weekly exercise minutes, or strength gains.

Achievability: Given your current situation, resources, and abilities, set challenging but realistic goals that are doable. To keep momentum and drive going, think about dividing more ambitious objectives into more doable benchmarks.

Relevance: Make sure your objectives line up with your priorities, values, and long-term dreams. Consider the significance of each goal for you and the ways in which completing them will improve your general health and standard of living.

Time-Bound: To instill a sense of urgency and accountability, set deadlines for each goal. Establish clear goals or dates to strive toward, but be adaptable and change course as needed to account for developments and unanticipated events.

Accountability and Support: You might want to discuss your objectives with a friend, relative, or fitness expert who can help hold you accountable and offer support as you go. Getting help from a professional or joining a community might also improve your path.

Setting SMART goals (Specific, Measurable, Achievable, Relevant, Time-Bound) and completing a thorough self-evaluation will help you get started on the right track toward health and fitness and increase your chances of success and long-term adherence. To keep your goals in line with your changing requirements and priorities, don't forget to evaluate and modify them on a frequent basis.

## Knowledge and comprehension

The cornerstones of any successful path to health and fitness are knowledge and education. Having information gives you the ability to set reasonable goals, make wise decisions, and maintain long-term healthy behaviors. Here are some ways to improve your knowledge and comprehension in this field:

Learn the fundamentals of basic anatomy and physiology to gain insight into the functioning of the human body's many systems (skeletal, muscular, and cardiovascular, for example) and how they interact with one another during exercise and physical activity.

The fundamentals of nutrition, such as macronutrients (carbohydrates, proteins, and fats), micronutrients (vitamins and minerals), and their functions in promoting general health and fitness objectives, should be understood.

Exercise Science: Gain knowledge about the various forms of exercise, including cardiovascular, strength, and flexibility training, as well as how they can enhance body composition, fitness levels, and general well-being.

# CHAPTER TWO

Training Principles: Recognize the fundamentals of training, such as overload, recuperation, specificity, and progression. Discover how to create training plans that work for you and are specific to your tastes, skills, and goals.

Injury Prevention and Safety: To reduce the chance of getting hurt while exercising, familiarize yourself with safe practices, effective exercise techniques, and injury prevention tactics.

Examine the psychological aspects of behavior modification, motivation, and the maintenance of healthy lifestyle choices. Recognize typical obstacles to change and effective ways to overcome them.

Stress Management and emotional Health: Discover how stress affects both your physical and emotional well-being, as well as effective stress-reduction, relaxation, and resilience-building strategies.

Acknowledge the significance of sleep and recuperation in enhancing physical well-being and overall efficiency. Recognize how length and quality of sleep impact metabolism, brain function, and post-exercise recovery, among other elements of health.

Health Screening and Risk Factors: Become knowledgeable about the significance of routine health screenings and check-ups as well as common health risk factors including diabetes, high blood pressure, and obesity.

Evidence-Based Practices: Keep up with the latest findings and recommendations in the areas of nutrition, exercise, and health. Sort fact from fiction by searching for reliable sources and critically assessing information sources.

Continuing Education: Make a commitment to lifelong learning and ongoing development by looking for educational opportunities, including online courses, workshops, seminars, and certifications in the fields of health and fitness.

By making an investment in your education and comprehension of health and fitness principles, you'll create a strong knowledge base that will support and mentor you as you work toward your objectives and lead a happy, healthy life.

## Creating Your Exercise Program

A personalized exercise plan must take into account your tastes, goals, level of fitness right now, and available funds. This is a step-by-step approach to assist you in designing a customized exercise program:

1. Establish Specific Objectives:

Establish quantifiable, precise objectives like losing weight, gaining muscle, improving cardiovascular health, or becoming more flexible.

To stay motivated and focused, set both short-
and long-term goals.

2. Determine Your Present State of Fitness:

Assess your body composition, muscular
strength, flexibility, and cardiovascular
endurance.

Think about any restrictions or injuries that
might affect the types of exercises you choose.

3. Select Pleasure-Seeking Activities:

Choose physical hobbies and workouts that you
truly enjoy, such as yoga, dance, weightlifting,
swimming, cycling, or jogging.

To keep your workouts engaging and avoid
monotony, mix things up.

4. Establish a Balanced Schedule:

To address various areas of fitness, incorporate a combination of strength training, flexibility training, and aerobic (cardiovascular) workouts.

Aim for 75 minutes of vigorous-intensity aerobic activity or at least 150 minutes of moderate-intensity aerobic activity per week, in addition to two or more days of muscle-strengthening activities.

5. Increase Intensity Gradually:

Increasing the resistance, duration, or intensity of your workouts gradually will allow you to overload them more and more.

Pay attention to your body and refrain from overexerting yourself, particularly if you're just starting out.

6. Plan Frequent Exercises:

Schedule a specific period of time each week for exercising.

Depending on your goals and availability, try to work out three to five times a week at the very least. Be consistent.

7. Include Recuperation and Rest:

In order to avoid overtraining and lower the chance of injury, give yourself enough time to relax and recover in between sessions.

On rest days, incorporate active recovery exercises like yoga, stretching, or walking.

8. Talk about Hydration and Nutrition:

Give your body the nutrition and energy it needs for activity and recuperation by eating well-balanced meals and snacks.

Drink plenty of water to stay hydrated, especially before, during, and after exercise.

9. Track Your Development:

Using a fitness notebook, app, or wearable gadget, keep track of your exercises, advancement, and accomplishments.

Regularly review your objectives and modify your exercise regimen in light of your development and personal preferences.

10. Seek Expert Advice When Necessary:

To create a personalized fitness program that meets your requirements and objectives, think about collaborating with a licensed personal trainer, fitness coach, or exercise physiologist.

If you have any medical issues or ailments that could need for specific advice, speak with a healthcare provider.

You can achieve long-lasting results and reap the rewards of better health and fitness by following these guidelines and creating a well-rounded fitness plan that suits your preferences and goals.

Developing a good diet is crucial to maintaining energy levels, exercise objectives, and general health. The following actions will assist you in creating and sustaining a sustainable, well-balanced approach to nutrition:

1. Recognize Your Nutritional Needs:

Discover the fundamentals of nutrition, including the functions of vitamins, minerals, and macronutrients (carbohydrates, proteins, and fats) in the body.

Recognize your unique nutritional requirements in light of your age, gender, activity level, and health objectives.

2. Emphasis on Complete, High-Nutrient Foods:

Give top priority to entire foods, including whole grains, legumes, nuts, seeds, and fruits and vegetables as well as lean proteins.

To guarantee a wide range of nutrients, try to incorporate a variety of vibrant fruits and vegetables into your meals.

3. Use Portion Control Techniques:

Keep an eye on portion sizes and steer clear of excessive amounts, particularly when it comes to high-calorie items.

To estimate the right serving sizes, use visual indicators like food scales, measuring cups, or hand-sized amounts.

4. Eat Often and Consciously:

Set aside regular times for meals, and try to consume a balanced diet that includes healthy fats, carbohydrates, and protein.

Slow down, chew your meal well, and pay attention to your body's signals of hunger and fullness to cultivate mindful eating.

5. Maintain Hydration:

Throughout the day, consume enough water to stay hydrated and support different body processes.

Avoid overindulging in sugary drinks and caffeine by substituting water, herbal teas, or infused water.

6. Arrange and Get Ready for Meals:

Spend some time organizing your weekly menu and snacks, making sure to include a range of wholesome items.

To save time and guarantee that healthier options are always available, batch cook and prepare meals in advance.

7. Pay Attention to Your Body:

Pay attention to your body's signals of hunger, fullness, and contentment instead of following rigid diet guidelines or outside stimuli.

In moderation, give in to your urges, and maintain balance and flexibility in your eating habits.

8. Eat Fewer Ultra-Processed and Processed Foods:

Reduce your consumption of highly processed meals that are heavy in unhealthy fats, added sugars, and artificial additives.

Whenever possible, go for whole, less processed options.

9. Seek Assistance and Responsibility:

Be in the company of friends, family, or peers who are as committed to their health and well-being as you are.

For individualized advice and assistance, think about consulting with a certified dietitian or nutritionist.

10. Practice Being Flexible and Self-Compassionate:

Recognize that developing good eating habits is a journey rather than a destination and treat yourself with kindness.

Accept flexibility and give yourself permission to occasionally indulge in sweets or delicacies without feeling guilty.

You may develop and sustain healthy eating habits that support your long-term fitness and general health objectives by adopting these methods into your daily life and continuously making decisions that put nourishment and well-being first.

Starting a journey toward better health and fitness can be very fulfilling, but it's not without difficulties and roadblocks. The following are some typical roadblocks you may run into and the solutions for them:

1. Absence of drive:

Method: Determine the significant reasons behind your wish to enhance your physical and mental well-being by discovering your "why". Envision the benefits reaching your objectives will bring to your life.

Take Action: Establish attainable objectives that are reasonable and divide them into smaller deadlines. Reward yourself for making progress to keep yourself inspired.

2. Time Restrictions:

Plan your exercise and meal preparation into your daily schedule like you would any other important appointment. This will help you prioritize your health.

Action: When time is tight, choose workouts that are shorter and more effective. Taking the stairs, walking or biking to work, or doing brief workouts at home are all great ways to include physical activity into your daily life.

3. Absence of Assistance:

Approach: Encircle yourself with a network of friends, family, or online groups that are all committed to the same levels of exercise and health.

Action: Tell those close to you about your needs and aspirations. Also, look for workout partners or accountability partners who can help you stay motivated and inspired.

4. Boredom or Stuckness:

Plan: Try different exercises, classes, or activities to keep your workouts fresh and exciting.

Take action: To keep yourself interested and motivated, set new objectives or tasks. Prioritize progress over perfection and acknowledge even the smallest accomplishments along the way.

5. Cravings or Emotional Eating:

Strategy: Recognize the situations that set off emotional eating episodes and create more positive coping strategies like journaling, mindfulness, or talking to friends.

Action: Eat mindfully and in moderation to prevent overindulging; keep wholesome snacks on hand to quell cravings.

6. Physical limitations or injuries:

Approach: Pay attention to your body and put safety before enduring discomfort. Adjust workouts or look for substitutes that accommodate your constraints.

Take action: For advice on correct form, preventing injuries, and rehabilitation activities, speak with a medical practitioner or physical therapist.

7. Impractical Expectations:

Strategy: Based on your unique abilities, resources, and lifestyle, set attainable, realistic goals.

Action: As you work toward your goals, remember to be patient with yourself and concentrate on making progress rather than perfection. Appreciate every small victory you get along the way.

8. Budgetary Restrictions:

Plan: Look for less expensive options, such bodyweight workouts, online training videos, or outdoor activities, in place of pricey gym subscriptions or equipment.

Take action: Look into local wellness programs, free exercise classes, and community resources. Invest in high-caliber, multifunctional household appliances.

9. Insufficient Information or Advice: Approach: Learn about the fundamentals of health and fitness from reliable sources like books, websites, or qualified experts.

Action: To get precise guidance, accountability, and support, think about collaborating with a personal trainer, dietitian, or health coach.

10. All-or-nothing thinking or perfectionism: strategy Be kind to yourself and accept that

imperfections are a necessary part of the journey. Instead of aiming for perfection, concentrate on consistency and forward motion.

Action: Be realistic with yourself and give yourself room to adjust to the ups and downs of life. Keep in mind that gradual, sustainable improvements over time can result in significant gains in fitness and health.

By identifying and resolving these common problems early on, you can avoid setbacks and continue on your path to improved health and fitness. Resilience, tenacity, and self-compassion are essential for long-term success.

# CHAPTER THREE

## Putting New Lifestyles Into Practice

On your journey to health and fitness, implementing lifestyle changes requires dedication, perseverance, and a readiness to make long-lasting changes to your daily routine. Here's how to successfully implement lifestyle modifications:

1. Start Small: To begin, identify one or two specific changes you would like to make, such increasing the amount of vegetables in your meals or taking a daily walk.

Prioritize the development of these new habits before gradually implementing other modifications.

2. Establish SMART goals: These are objectives that are Time-bound, Relevant, Measurable, Achievable, and Specific.

As an illustration, make an effort to exercise for thirty minutes five days a week or to consume eight glasses of water each day.

3. Make Consistency a Priority: Developing new behaviors requires consistency. Make a commitment to consistently doing the tasks you have chosen, particularly on days when you lack motivation.

To assist you keep on track, establish accountability systems, rituals, or reminders.

4. Create a Support Network: Assist and inspire yourself on your path to better health and fitness by surrounding yourself with friends, family, or peers.

To meet people who share your interests, think about signing up for a support group, fitness class, or online community.

5. Concentrate on Progress Rather than Perfection: Accept the process and acknowledge that obstacles are a normal part of the journey.

Honor your growth and accomplishments, no matter how small, and don't be too harsh on yourself when you have setbacks.

6. Plan and Prepare: Make sure your weekly schedule includes workouts, meal prep sessions, and other healthful activities. Plan ahead.

To curb impulsive eating, have wholesome snacks readily accessible and stock your kitchen with wholesome foods.

7. Make Nutrient-Dense Food Selections: Try to incorporate a variety of nutrient-dense foods, such as fruits, vegetables, whole grains, lean meats, and healthy fats, into your meals.

By observing your body's signals of hunger and fullness and savoring every bite, you can practice mindful eating.

8. Be Active Throughout the Day: Try to incorporate physical activity into your daily

schedule by doing things like walking or biking to work, climbing stairs, or performing housework.

To keep your body moving, use brief movement breaks to break up extended periods of sitting.

9. Control Stress and Make Sleep a Priority:

To improve relaxation and mental health, try stress-reduction techniques like yoga, meditation, or deep breathing.

Aim for seven to nine hours of good sleep every night to aid in healing and general well-being.

10. Have Patience and Persistence: Keep in mind that it takes time for new lifestyle choices to become deeply ingrained habits. Even when things seem to be moving slowly toward your

goals, have patience with yourself and never give up.

Remain mindful of the long-term benefits of your work and have faith that persistent effort will eventually pay off.

By adopting these small, consistent lifestyle adjustments, you'll lay the groundwork for lifelong improvements in your general well-being, fitness, and health.

## Monitoring Development and Modifying Approaches

Any effective path to health and fitness must include monitoring progress and modifying techniques. Here's how to effectively track your development and make the necessary corrections as you go:

1. Define measures and Goals: To monitor your progress, set up quantifiable, clear measures like weight, body measurements, fitness assessments, or performance enhancements.

Establish definite short- and long-term objectives that align with your objectives and intended results.

2. Select Monitoring Techniques:

To continuously track your progress, use a variety of tracking tools, including wearable technology, spreadsheets, journals, and fitness applications.

Regularly record relevant information, such as exercises, nutrition intake, measurements, and self-reported emotional state.

3. Monitor Crucial Indices:

Keep an eye on vital indicators of your health and fitness, like your flexibility, strength gains, cardiovascular endurance, body weight, and body composition (such as body fat percentage).

Keep an eye on other factors that affect your health, such as your energy, mood, quality of sleep, and general contentment with your way of life.

4. Regularly Evaluate Your Progress:

Set up frequent checkpoints to track your development and assess if you're getting closer to your objectives.

Think back on the things that are working well and any areas that might require improvement.

5. Celebrate Your Success: No matter how small your victory may have been, give it your due. Acknowledge the time and energy you have invested in your path.

To stay motivated, treat yourself to non-food rewards or have a family and friend celebration of your accomplishments.

6. Identify Challenges and Barriers: Take note of any issues or impediments to your development, such as deadlines, a lack of drive, or plateaus.

Be truthful with yourself about the areas in which you might need additional help or resources to get over obstacles.

7. Modify Approaches Consequently:

Determine what elements of your exercise routine, eating habits, or lifestyle choices may need change based on your progress evaluation.

Try other strategies including changing your diet, getting guidance from a specialist, or changing your exercise regimen.

8. Remain Adaptive and Flexible: Have the flexibility to change your plan of action in response to input from your body and your outcomes. Adopt a growth mindset and see obstacles as chances to improve and learn.

Keep an open mind and look into novel approaches, pastimes, or dietary plans that can better support your objectives.

9. Ask for Help and Take Accountability:

Assist yourself by interacting with a mentor, coach, or encouraging group that may offer guidance, reinforcement, and responsibility.

Talk about your goals, failures, and successes with people who can encourage you and hold you responsible.

10. Remain Committed to the Process: Recognize that obstacles are a normal part of the process and that development may not always be linear. Hold fast to your beliefs and your aims throughout the process.

Recall that maintaining your health and fitness over the long run requires commitment and consistency.

You will be more prepared to overcome obstacles and stay on track to achieving your health and fitness objectives if you routinely assess your progress, identify areas for improvement, and modify your approaches.

## Honoring Success and Keeping the Fire Going

Maintaining momentum and celebrating accomplishments are crucial components of staying motivated and making progress on your path to improved health and fitness. Here are some suggestions to keep you inspired and able to appreciate your accomplishments:

1. Acknowledge Your Achievements: No matter how small, take the time to acknowledge and enjoy each milestone and accomplishment. Recognize your accomplishments, no matter if they involve sticking to your training schedule, achieving a fitness goal, or making better dietary choices.

2. Take Stock of Your Journey: Take stock of your progress since you began your path to better health and fitness. Recall the challenges you've surmounted, the habits you've changed, and the advancements you've achieved. Make the most of this reflection as motivation to keep going.

3. Reward Yourself: Give yourself incentives or rewards when you reach milestones or accomplish objectives. This may be a massage, new workout gear, or a day off to relax and rejuvenate something you've been wanting for a while.

4. Celebrate Your Success: Let your loved ones, friends, and support system know what you've accomplished. Sharing your victories with others can increase your sense of fulfillment and achievement. It also enables you to encourage and uplift others as they embark on their own fitness and health journeys.

5. Track Your Progress: Whether it's via photos, journaling, or tracking metrics, make sure you have a record of your accomplishments. Having

tangible proof of your accomplishments can boost your self-esteem and serve as a helpful reminder of your progress.

6. create New Objectives: To keep pushing yourself and maintain momentum, create new objectives after acknowledging your accomplishments. These objectives may pertain to your nutrition, exercise regimen, or other aspects of your overall health. Ascertain that they are time-bound, relevant, quantifiable, attainable, and specified (SMART).

7. Accept Non-Scale Victories: Honor non-scale achievements like heightened confidence, higher energy, happier moods, or better sleep. These accomplishments are frequently markers of general health and well-being and are as

significant to weight or body composition changes.

8. Remain Consistent: Maintaining momentum on your path to health and fitness requires consistency. Follow through on your commitments and routines even on the days when you don't feel motivated. Keep in mind that small, regular acts add up over time.

9. Find Joy in the Process: Try not to get too caught up in the destination and instead concentrate on having fun along the way. Discover hobbies you enjoy, experiment with new diets and exercise regimens, and accept the process of growth and development in yourself.

10. Practice Gratitude: Make an effort to be grateful for your body's potential, other people's support, and the chance to pursue fitness and health. Developing an attitude of gratitude might help you stay motivated in challenging situations.

11. Remain Inspired: Take a cue from people who have accomplished similar feats or surmounted comparable obstacles. Join online forums, read success stories, and follow fitness influencers to get support and motivation.

You'll be more prepared to maintain momentum and advance toward health and fitness if you recognize your accomplishments, set new goals, practice consistency, and enjoy the ride. Remind yourself to cherish every step forward, no matter how small, and to be patient with yourself.

## CONCLUSION

In conclusion, achieving physical, mental, and emotional well-being is a profoundly personal and life-changing event that is your road to health and fitness. You have built the foundation for long-lasting change and development by embracing the concepts of self-awareness, goal-setting, and ongoing learning throughout this journey.

You've overcome obstacles, experienced triumphs, and welcomed the ups and downs of the journey. You've made amazing progress toward enhancing your overall quality of life, fitness level, and health by commitment, consistency, and tenacity.

As you think back on your journey, keep in mind that living a balanced, resilient, and self-care lifestyle is just as important as reaching your destination. Maintain your focus on your health, pay attention to your body, and cultivate habits that promote both your mental and physical well-being.

Continue establishing new objectives, taking on fresh difficulties, and taking pleasure in the journey. Embrace the company of people and communities that encourage and inspire you to be the best version of yourself.

Above all, keep in mind that your quest for health and fitness is a never-ending adventure of empowerment, advancement, and self-discovery. Accept each day with love, compassion, and commitment, understanding that each step you take will get you one step closer to leading a full and active life.

Your journey to health and fitness may take you anywhere you want to go as long as you have faith in your own abilities and a dedication to lifetime healthy. Continue moving forward, one step at a time, and have faith that your path has the ability to completely change not just your body but also your mind, spirit, and entire existence.

THE END